HERBAL ANTIVIRAL SUPPORT

Empower Your Immune System, Explore The Healing Potential Of Resilient Well-Being

DR. JEREMY ALLEY

Copyright © DR. JEREMY ALLEY 2024

All rights reserved. No part of this publication may be reproduced, distributed, or transmitted in any form or by any means, including photocopying, recording, or other electronic or mechanical methods, without the prior written permission of the author, except in the case of brief quotations embodied in critical reviews and certain other noncommercial uses permitted by copyright law.

Disclaimer:

The information provided in this book, is intended for general informational purposes only and should not be considered as professional advice.

The author has made every effort to ensure the accuracy of the information presented. However, readers are advised to consult with a qualified healthcare professional before attempting any herbal remedies or making significant changes to their wellness routine. Individual health conditions vary, and what may be suitable for one person may not be appropriate for another.

It is important to note that the author is not in any endorsement deal, partnership, or affiliation with any organization, brand, or company mentioned in this book. Any references to specific products or services are based on the author's personal experience or general knowledge and do not imply an endorsement or promotion of those products or services.

Contents

Introduction

The investigation of complementary and alternative methods to boost the immune system has drawn a lot of attention in the field of health and wellness. Using the long history of medical plant use, herbal antiviral support is a promising way to strengthen the body's defenses against viral infections. This talk explores the role of herbal remedies in antiviral support, looking at their historical origins, current applicability, and growing popularity among those looking for natural substitutes for traditional pharmaceutical treatments.

The Value of Herbal Antiviral Assistance

It is impossible to exaggerate the value of herbal antiviral assistance, particularly in a society where viral infections present serious health risks. Because herbal medicines can boost immunity and lessen the effects of viral diseases, they have been used for centuries in a variety of cultures. This section delves into the rationale for the increasing demand for herbal antiviral assistance. These rationales include the allure of natural therapies, the pursuit of preventative measures, and the aim to reduce the adverse effects linked to pharmaceutical interventions.

Herbs that Have Antiviral Effects

This section takes the reader on a tour of the wide range of medicinal plants, highlighting important herbs that have strong antiviral effects. Every plant, including licorice root, astragalus, and echinacea, has a different combination of chemicals that let them work as antivirals. People can choose wisely when to add these herbs to their wellness regimens by being aware of their historical applications and modes of action.

Science Underpinnings of Herbal Antiviral Activity

This section explores the scientific basis of herbal antiviral action, explaining how the bioactive chemicals found in medicinal herbs work to fight viral infections. Examining studies and study results offers a thorough grasp of how these herbs affect immune system function, prevent virus multiplication, and have antiviral properties. This scientific viewpoint gives the conventional wisdom about herbal medicines more nuance.

Support for Herbal Antivirals in Traditional Medicine

Herbal treatments have long been used by traditional medical systems throughout the world to treat a range of illnesses, including viral infections. This section delves into the historical foundations of herbal antiviral assistance in conventional treatments, including Indigenous healing systems, Traditional Chinese Medicine, and Ayurveda. The tried-and-true effectiveness of herbal remedies can be better understood by looking at the cultural settings and wisdom that are ingrained in these methods.

Combining Traditional and Modern Medicine

The integration of herbal antiviral assistance with traditional medical treatments has gained recognition in the pursuit of holistic healthcare. This section looks at the possible interactions between antiviral drugs and herbal medicines, highlighting situations where using both together could result in better therapeutic outcomes. The examination of cooperative initiatives between herbalists and medical experts highlights how integrated medicine is changing.

Safety and Things to Think About

Although herbal therapies provide an all-natural means of providing antiviral assistance, caution about safety and possible interactions must be taken into account. This section explores the significance of using informational medicine, going into topics including dose, possible adverse effects, and contraindications. Encouraging people to take responsibly sourced herbal supplements is essential to guaranteeing the effectiveness and security of these natural remedies.

The investigation of herbal antiviral support highlights the diverse range of natural therapies that can be utilized to promote optimal immune function. This discussion guides anyone looking for a well-rounded and knowledgeable approach to antiviral assistance, including everything from the scientific understanding of herbal activities to the historical foundations of traditional medicine. The convergence of traditional and modern medicine offers the possibility of integrative solutions, which open the door to a customized and comprehensive approach to immune well-being.

CHAPTER ONE

RECOGNISING VIRUSES

Viruses are little infectious organisms that are limited to replicating only within the live cells of their host. Viruses do not possess the cellular machinery required for autonomous life, in contrast to bacteria. They are made up of genetic material, either RNA or DNA, encased in a capsid, a protein covering. Developing practical methods to counteract the negative effects of viruses on health requires an understanding of their nature.

Describe Viruses.

Viruses can have single- or double-stranded genetic material, and they can be of different sizes and forms. One reason viruses can infect so many different types of hosts—humans, animals, plants, and even bacteria—is their diversity. Humans frequently contract viruses that cause the flu, the common cold, and more serious illnesses like

COVID-19. The evolution of viruses makes it difficult to create effective antiviral therapies.

The Transmission Of Viruses

Viruses use several techniques to transfer from one host to another. For instance, respiratory viruses are frequently transmitted by respiratory droplets released during coughing, sneezing, or talking by an infected individual. Certain viruses spread through direct contact with bodily fluids, whereas others are disseminated by infected surfaces or fomites. Comprehending these pathways of transmission is essential for putting preventative measures into action and creating antiviral tactics.

Viruses' Effect On Health

Human health can be significantly impacted by viruses, ranging from minor ailments to serious, life-threatening conditions. The body's defense against viral infections is largely dependent on the immune system, but many viruses can elude the immune system or trigger an overreaction that damages the immune system. The development of antiviral therapies targeted at lowering the morbidity and mortality connected to viral infections is aided by continuing research on the effects of viruses on health.

Herbal Antiviral Assistance

For millennia, traditional medical systems have employed herbs as cures for a wide range of illnesses, including viral infections. Even though the research of antiviral drugs has advanced significantly in modern medicine, interest in investigating the potential of herbal antiviral support is developing. Numerous herbs have antiviral bioactive components that can be utilized as preventative measures or as a supplement to traditional treatments.

Herbs That Have Antiviral Effects

In vitro studies have shown the antiviral properties of some plants. Ginger, licorice root, garlic, echinacea, and elderberries are a few examples. These herbs include substances called flavonoids, polyphenols, and alkaloids that, by obstructing virus reproduction, entrance into host cells, or immune response modulation, exhibit antiviral actions. The precise mechanisms of action of these natural substances are still being researched.

Safety And Effectiveness Of Herbal Antiviral Therapy

Although many people consider herbal medicines to be natural and safe, it's important to assess their effectiveness and safety about antiviral support. The caliber and structure of scientific research on the efficacy of herbal remedies against particular viruses varies. Ensuring the safe use of herbal antiviral support requires an understanding of the right dosage, possible side effects, and combinations with conventional drugs.

Combining Traditional Antiviral Treatments With Integration

In the medical world, there is interest in combining traditional antiviral treatments with herbal antiviral assistance.

According to certain research, taking herbal medicines along with prescription antivirals may increase their effectiveness or lower the possibility of drug resistance.

To create precise criteria for the safe and efficient combination of conventional antiviral medicines and herbal remedies, more research is necessary.

Points To Remember When Using

People should speak with healthcare providers before adding herbal antiviral assistance to their routine, particularly if they are currently on prescription drugs. Individuals who are expecting or nursing, as well as those with underlying medical concerns, should use caution and consult with healthcare professionals.

To maximize the advantages and minimize the hazards of herbal treatments, it is important to understand their proper use and potential interactions.

Herbal antiviral support offers an intriguing field for research in the quest for holistic approaches to health. Herbs have the potential to be beneficial in the battle against viral infections, but it's important to use them responsibly, taking into account medical specialists' advice, specific health circumstances, and scientific data. Our capacity to fight viral illnesses may be improved by further investigation into the antiviral qualities of herbs and how they might be used with traditional treatments.

CHAPTER TWO

WHAT IS HERBAL MEDICINE'S BASIS?

Because of its possible antiviral qualities, herbal medicine, an age-old technique with roots in traditional healing systems, has attracted increased attention recently.

The application of plant-based therapies to enhance the body's natural processes is emphasized in this holistic approach to health. For people looking for complementary and alternative approaches to treating viral infections, it is essential to comprehend the fundamentals of herbal medicine.

Overview Of Herbal Medicine

A wide variety of plants are used in herbal medicine, and each one has special chemicals that add to its medicinal properties. For millennia, people have relied on the medicinal qualities of plants to treat a variety of illnesses. Civilizations all over the world have used herbs to treat various problems.

Herbal therapies are thought to strengthen the immune system, prevent viral replication, and lessen infection-related symptoms when used in conjunction with antiviral therapy.

The Effects Of Herbs On The Body

Herbs affect several physiological systems in the body through a variety of interactions. Alkaloids, flavonoids, and terpenes are a few examples of the bioactive substances found in many herbs that give them their therapeutic qualities.

When it comes to antiviral assistance, certain herbs work directly against viruses by preventing them from attaching to or replicating, while other herbs boost immunity to strengthen the body's defenses.

Comprehending these mechanisms is essential to fully using herbal treatments.

Safety And Precautions

Although herbal medicine shows promise in providing antiviral support, it is important to practice caution when using it. Proper dosage, possible drug interactions, and the need to speak with a healthcare provider before introducing herbal therapies into a person's routine are all safety concerns.

It is crucial to be aware of the potential hazards associated with particular herbs as they may trigger negative reactions in certain people. When contemplating herbal therapies, those who are pregnant, nursing, or have pre-existing medical issues should take extra precautions and consult a professional.

A framework for investigating the possibilities of plant-based therapies in antiviral support is provided by the fundamentals of herbal therapy. The importance of this all-encompassing approach to health is highlighted by the lengthy history of herbal medicine and our growing knowledge of the physiological interactions between herbs and the body.

To maximize the advantages of herbal antiviral support, however, a careful and knowledgeable approach is required, which includes paying attention to safety concerns and seeking professional advice.

CHAPTER THREE

ESSENTIAL HERBS FOR SUPPORTING AGAINST

Herbal therapies for antiviral support have drawn a lot of attention because of their potential to strengthen the body's natural defenses against viral infections.

Of all the herbs known to have antiviral qualities, Echinacea is nature's immune system builder. Native American societies have long used this herb, which is widely distributed in North America, to strengthen their immune systems.

Because of its active ingredients, flavonoids, and alkamides, which are thought to have immune-modulating properties, echinacea is a well-liked option for people looking for natural antiviral support.

Nature's Immune System Booster: Echinacea

Because it can increase the generation and activity of white blood cells, which are essential for the body's fight against infections, echinacea is known for being a potent immune booster.

The plant is frequently used to lessen the intensity and length of respiratory illnesses, such as colds. Echinacea is accessible for a variety of tastes because it comes in tinctures, capsules, and teas, among other forms.

Elderberry: A Strong Herbal Antiviral

Elderberry is another well-known herb for antiviral assistance. Elderberries, prized for their abundance of antioxidants, have been used for ages to ward off colds and the flu.

Flavonoids found in the deep purple berries of the Elder tree may help stop viruses from entering cells and stop them from replicating. Elderberry teas, syrups, and pills are easily found and offer a handy method to include this powerful antiviral plant in one's daily regimen.

The Natural Antibiotic Of Garlic

Known as "nature's antibiotic," garlic has been shown to possess antibacterial qualities, including antiviral capabilities.

Garlic contains a sulfur-containing chemical called allicin, which is thought to have antiviral and immune-stimulating properties. Historically, garlic has been used to prevent infections and promote respiratory health.

Taking supplements containing fresh garlic or including it in one's diet may enhance overall antiviral support.

Andrographis: An Effective Herbal Antiviral

Native to South Asian nations, Andrographis is becoming more well-known for its powerful antiviral qualities. Andrographolides, which are found in the herb, are thought to have immune-stimulating and antiviral properties.

Andrographis has long been used to treat respiratory infections and may also help lessen the intensity and course of viral infections. For people looking for natural antiviral protection, Andrographis-containing supplements and herbal formulations are becoming more and more popular.

Using herbal medicines to assist the immune system against viruses provides a comprehensive approach to immune system reinforcement.

Andrographis, Garlic, Elderberry, and Echinacea are a few of the plants that nature has provided as a defense against viral diseases.

Including these herbs in one's wellness regimen, either through food or supplements, may strengthen immunity and promote general health.

Before beginning a new herbal regimen, as with any health-related decision, it is best to speak with a healthcare provider, particularly for people who are on medication or have pre-existing medical conditions.

CHAPTER FOUR

MANUFACTURING HERBAL CURE

Using the power of different medicinal plants to strengthen the body's immune system and fight viral infections is the process of making herbal medications for antiviral assistance. For ages, traditional medical systems have employed this all-encompassing method, which is still a beneficial choice for people looking for natural substitutes for prescription antiviral drugs.

Herbal Teas To Promote Antiviral Effects

One well-liked and easily available option to include antiviral herbs in your daily routine is through herbal teas.

Herbal teas derived from plants like ginger, elderberry, and echinacea have long been used to strengthen immunity and ward against illness. Elderberry possesses antiviral and anti-inflammatory qualities, whereas echinacea is particularly recognized for its ability to strengthen the immune system. The anti-inflammatory and antioxidant qualities of ginger give these teas a comforting, cozy quality.

Herbal Extracts And Tinctures

Concentrated versions of therapeutic plants, such as herbal tinctures and extracts, can be effective companions in the fight against viruses.

Glycerites have glycerin as their foundation, whereas tinctures are usually extracts made with alcohol. A few antiviral herbs that are frequently used in tinctures are olive leaf, astragalus, and licorice root. Astragalus is well known for its immune-modulating qualities, and licorice root has been investigated for its antiviral capabilities. Compounds in olive leaf extract have antiviral properties, which makes it a useful addition to herbal tinctures.

Homemade Herbal Syrups

Making your herbal syrups is a delicious and practical method to take antiviral herbs. Thyme, oregano, and honey are a few immune-boosting herbs that can be used to make syrups.

Herbal syrups benefit greatly from the antiviral and antibacterial qualities of thyme and oregano. Apart from its ability to sweeten, honey has been utilized for its antibacterial and calming characteristics.

 By combining these herbs in a syrup, you can boost the flavor and make a powerful antiviral cure.

Herbal treatments provide a wide array of choices for anyone looking for all-natural antiviral assistance.

 Incorporating herbal treatments, such as tinctures, syrups, or teas, into your wellness routine can support immunological health in general.

While herbs may be helpful, it's important to remember that you should always speak with a healthcare provider, particularly if you have underlying medical concerns or are taking other medications.

CHAPTER FIVE

INCLUDING HERBS IN EVERYDAY LIFE

Including herbs in daily life can be a comprehensive way to support general health and well-being, especially in terms of antiviral support.

Because of their potential therapeutic benefits, traditional medical systems all over the world have utilized herbs for ages. Including herbs in every facet of everyday life—from cooking to taking supplements—can support a holistic approach to well-being.

Including Herbs In Your Nutrition

By including herbs in your regular diet, you can take advantage of one of the easiest methods to utilize their antiviral properties. Herbs with antiviral and immune-boosting qualities include garlic, ginger, and turmeric.

Adding these herbs to food improves its flavor and provides a natural barrier against viruses. Adding herbs to your food in inventive ways can make it tasty and healthy, whether you use them in salads or soups.

Herbal Supplements For Extended Assistance

Herbal pills, in addition to adding herbs to meals regularly, can provide sustained immune system support. Herbs with possible antiviral qualities that are frequently taken as supplements include astragalus, echinacea, and elderberry.

These supplements are frequently offered in a range of forms, such as tinctures, teas, and capsules.

Utilizing these herbal supplements on a regular and consistent basis may strengthen the body's defenses against viral infections, offering a preventative method of maintaining good health.

Developing herbal remedies that strengthen the immune system can be a fun and useful strategy to improve antiviral support.

Teas prepared from immune-stimulating herbs, such as thyme, licorice, and echinacea, can have calming and healthful effects.

Furthermore, utilizing herbs in homemade syrups or infusing them into honey offers a delicious and nutritious substitute for store-bought products. Personalized immune support can be achieved by experimenting with different herbal combinations in recipes, which can be tailored to meet the needs and preferences of each individual.

Using herbs to their full potential requires a multimodal strategy that includes recipe development, supplementation, and cooking techniques. Even though each person reacts to herbs differently, incorporating these organic materials into daily living might help create a more thorough antiviral support plan. Before adding new herbs or supplements to one's regimen, it is best to speak with a healthcare provider, especially if one is taking medication or has pre-existing medical conditions.

CHAPTER SIX

ANTIVIRAL HERBAL SUPPORT FOR PARTICULAR CONDITIONS

For millennia, people have turned to herbal medicines to promote health and well-being. Certain herbs have demonstrated potential in offering antiviral support for particular circumstances when it comes to viral infections.

This section examines the potential advantages and drawbacks of using herbal medicines for common viral illnesses including the flu and cold.

Herbal Treatments For The Flu And Cold

Among the most common viral diseases, the cold and the flu can be uncomfortable and interfere with day-to-day activities.

Herbal treatments provide a safe and effective means of symptom relief and bolstering the body's defenses against illnesses. For example, echinacea has long been used to strengthen immunity, while elderberry has demonstrated antiviral qualities that may help lessen the intensity and length of cold and flu symptoms.

Herbs like licorice root and ginger can also help with symptoms like coughing and sore throat that are brought on by these viral infections.

To maximize the effectiveness of these herbal treatments in treating cold and flu symptoms, it is essential to understand the appropriate dosage and type.

Antiviral Assistance For Respiratory Well-Being

Coronaviruses and influenza are examples of respiratory viruses that frequently attack the respiratory system, producing symptoms like coughing, dyspnea, and soreness in the chest. Support from herbal antivirals can help to keep the respiratory system healthy and reduce these symptoms.

Due to their antibacterial qualities, herbs like peppermint, thyme, and oregano may be able to help fight respiratory viruses. Respiratory symptoms can be alleviated by inhaling essential oils that are extracted from these herbs, either through diffusers or steam. Additionally, the respiratory system can be soothed by herbal teas with substances like mullein and eucalyptus, which can help with comfort during viral infections.

Boosting The Immune System In The Event Of Virus Outbreaks

The body needs a strong immune system to fight off viral invaders. During viral outbreaks, herbal treatments can help strengthen the immune system by functioning as organic defenses against infections. For example, astragalus has long been utilized in Chinese medicine to support healthy immunological function.

Adding herbs that are known to help the body adapt to stress, like holy basil and ashwagandha, can be especially helpful when there is a viral outbreak and stress levels may be higher. Garlic and echinacea, two immune-boosting herbs, can also strengthen the body's defenses against several viral illnesses.

Herbal antiviral support provides a comprehensive and all-natural method of treating certain ailments including the flu and cold, enhancing respiratory health, and bolstering the immune system during viral epidemics. Even while these treatments can be beneficial additions to general health routines, it is crucial to seek the assistance of medical professionals for specific guidance, particularly in cases of severe or recurrent viral infections.

CHAPTER SEVEN

PRACTICES FOR LIFESTYLE ANTIVIRAL RESILIENCE

Sustaining a strong immune system and offering antiviral support hinges on leading a healthy lifestyle. Numerous holistic methods can improve general health and strengthen the body's defenses against viral infections.

Decreased Stress And Enhanced Immunity

Stress management is an essential component of antiviral assistance. Prolonged stress can impair immunity, increasing the body's vulnerability to viral infections.

Deep breathing exercises, mindfulness, and other stress-reduction methods can help lessen the negative effects of stress on immunological function.

Additionally, cultivating a positive outlook and discovering constructive coping mechanisms for life's setbacks can enhance general well-being. In addition to being good for mental health, chronic stress management is essential for a strong immune system.

Sleep's Function In Antiviral Support

An additional essential component in bolstering the body's antiviral defenses is getting enough good sleep.

The body goes through crucial immunological-related processes while you sleep, like producing cytokines and activating immune cells. These functions can be hampered by inadequate or poor-quality sleep, which increases the body's vulnerability to viral infections.

Antiviral support includes establishing a regular sleep schedule, furnishing a cozy sleeping space, and adhering to proper sleep hygiene. As part of a comprehensive wellness strategy, making sleep a priority can greatly support immune system health.

Physical Activity And Immunity

It is well-recognized that regular exercise strengthens the immune system and builds antiviral resilience. Exercise enhances cardiovascular health, boosts immune cell circulation, and aids in stress management—all of which are critical components in the prevention of viral infections.

Moderate-intensity exercise, such as jogging, cycling, or brisk walking, has been shown to have a favorable effect on immunological function. Striking a balance is crucial, though, as prolonged or vigorous activity may momentarily weaken the immune system.

A comprehensive and long-lasting fitness regimen is essential for achieving the immune-stimulating effects of physical activity.

Antiviral support can be greatly increased by embracing lifestyle choices that emphasize stress reduction, placing a high value on getting enough sleep and fitting regular exercise into daily schedules.

These all-encompassing methods build the groundwork for a healthier and more robust existence by improving immunological function as well as general well-being.

CHAPTER EIGHT

UNITING HERBAL AND CONVENTIONAL APPROACHES

The use of herbal treatments in conventional therapy has garnered considerable attention in the pursuit of efficacious antiviral support. The combination of these two strategies may boost the immune system as a whole and lead to better therapeutic results.

A more thorough and all-encompassing approach to treating viral infections may be experienced by those who combine the benefits of both conventional and herbal medicine.

Combining Herbs And Traditional Medicine

The strategic use of plant-based medicines in conjunction with conventional medical treatments is known as herbal antiviral support. The possible antiviral qualities of herbs such as astragalus, elderberry, and echinacea have been researched. Including these herbs in a treatment regimen can enhance the effects of prescription medications and provide a comprehensive defense against viral infections. Approaching integration with care, however, requires taking possible interactions into account and making sure that it is compatible with continuing medical measures.

Speaking With Medical Experts

It is important to consult medical authorities before starting any natural antiviral program. Herbs can provide beneficial assistance, but they can also worsen underlying medical issues or interfere with prescribed medications.

Healthcare providers—physicians, pharmacists, and herbalists—are essential in helping people incorporate herbal therapies into their overall healthcare plan safely and efficiently. Transparent communication guarantees that possible hazards are reduced and the selected herbs complement the person's unique medical requirements.

Case Studies And Triumphant Narratives

Analyzing case studies and success stories offers important insights into how herbal antiviral support is used in practice.

These real-world instances show how people have effectively managed and recovered from viral infections by combining herbal therapies with conventional medicine. Knowing about these situations might help people make well-informed decisions about using herbs in their personal care regimens. Success stories also provide insight into the possible advantages and difficulties of using herbal interventions, providing a practical assessment of their suitability in a range of circumstances.

CONCLUSION

Herbal antiviral support provides a comprehensive and all-natural method of enhancing health. For individuals contemplating alternate approaches to immune system support, the scientific validation of essential herbs and their potential antiviral capabilities offers insightful information. Herbs can support antiviral health, but it's important to use them wisely, cautiously, and in cooperation with medical professionals.

This synopsis highlights the key lessons learned from the herbal antiviral support conversation. Important topics include the background of herbal treatments in history, the scientific proof of the antiviral qualities of some herbs, and suggestions for responsible and safe use. Comprehending these pivotal aspects enables individuals to make knowledgeable choices about the integration of herbal treatments into their comprehensive well-being approach.

Encouraging Readers to Practice Antiviral Wellbeing

The final purpose of this investigation is to arm readers with information and comprehension regarding herbal antiviral support. By offering details on the workings, important herbs, supporting data from science, and factors to take into account, readers will be better equipped to make decisions that will improve their antiviral health. This empowerment promotes a health-focused strategy that combines conventional knowledge with new scientific discoveries to take a comprehensive and preventative approach to viral dangers.